INTRODUCTION TO
MOHS CRYOTOMY

Steven Lee

Trainer and Lecturer
Florida Licensed Histology Supervisor
HT ASCP since 1984
Certified by the American Society
of Mohs Histotechnologists

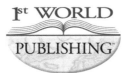

1st WORLD
PUBLISHING

Introduction to MOHS Cryotomy

Steven Lee

© Steven Lee 2006

Published by 1stWorld Publishing
1100 North 4th St. Fairfield, Iowa 52556
tel: 641-209-5000 • fax: 641-209-3001
web: www.1stworldpublishing.com

First Edition

LCCN: 2006903322
SoftCover B&W ISBN: 1-59540-882-7
SoftCover ISBN: 1-59540-864-9
HardCover ISBN: 1-59540-866-5
eBook ISBN: 1-59540-865-7

This material has been written and published solely for educational purposes. The author and the publisher shall have neither liability or responsibility to any person or entity with respect to any loss, damage or injury caused or alleged to be caused directly or indirectly by the information contained in this book.

TABLE OF CONTENTS

INTRODUCTION

A comprehensive course of study that is specifically designed to train the novice or the experienced Histotech in the art and science of Mohs Cryotomy. The need and demand for Mohs histotechs continues to increase, as more and more surgeons are recognizing the need and benefits to their patients, when they can offer this modality of treatment. As you become more and more proficient in this technique, your value to your employer will increase exponentially! This course of study will cover every detail that my 20 plus years of work in this field has taught me.

Your attention to everything taught and shown you, will enable you to market your skill to virtually any Mohs surgeon in the entire nation (except Rhode Island, where a Histology license is required).

Furthermore, my research has shown me that there is no course offered in the United States, that focuses this much time and energy, solely on the specialty of, 'Mohs Cryotomy'.

The time spent on each step of the process, will be largely dependent on you. This again, stresses the importance in your ability to be focused and organized. Some steps will come easier to you than others. Don't let yourself get too upset about it.

Working with you one on one, will be the, 'best teacher,' and you'll do very well. Speed, accuracy, organizational skills, the ability to focus and concentrate, are all vital to your success in Mohs cryotomy. The surgeon will at some point, *count on you, to help him feel without question, that the ease in which he was able to make his diagnosis and 'clear his patient', was directly related to your skill(s) as a Mohs histotech.*

Let me also say, that this manual could not possibly cover every single detail, that will be covered by those of you that have decided to take this course. Many times, you'll feel that I may sound very repetitive, in the things I will say and show to you..I promise you, it will only benefit you later. Practice, in this field is of great importance, so that you're able to build not just your confidence, but the speed at which you're able to process the specimens you receive. The faster (and of course, accurate) you become, the more value you'll have in your Mohs surgeons' eyes. More value to your boss, earns more money for you.

Need I say more?

Be sure you take notes during this course because there is that famous Law in life, known as 'Murphy's Law,' which basically says, that if something can go wrong, it will. I can't count the days in any given week, that I'm not challenged, in one way or the other, in this field.

The next page is going to give you a synopsis of the areas that we're going to cover, as we go through this subject matter together.

Remember, everything I tell you is not here, in print. Look at this manual as an overview of the areas we'll be covering.

Course Curriculum

1. Logging in of specimen

2. Slide Labeling

3. Maping and Inking of Specimen

4. Dissection

5. Chuck Preparation/Embedding of Specimen

6. Microtomy

7. Fixation

8. Staining

9. Coverslipping

10. Record Keeping

11. Equipment Maintenance

Logging In of Specimens

You will invariably find me repeating myself when I tell you that accuracy, is one of the most critical aspects of this work. Writing the *last name first*, *followed by the first name in the Mohs logbook* is where you'll begin.

Be sure you've copied the name exactly.

You would be amazed at the number of patients with the same and/or similar names. The difference in <u>one letter</u>, can cause all kinds of confusion, especially if the Dr. or an Inspector wishes to review a case at some later date.

Next of course, is logging in the <u>DATE</u> and following that, you'll be writing <u>case</u> numbers in your log book and ONLY you, will be logging in the <u>CASE NUMBER.</u> *Be sure that you transcribe your number(s) correctly.*

Try and imagine the nightmare of pre-labeling your logbook, only to realize days, weeks, or even months later, that you wrote the same number twice, causing you to re-label and correct, every single slide, laboratory record and patients' files. If an Inspector were to find the error that you missed, WATCH OUT!! Your boss will not be too happy with the possible consequences that he could face.

TYPICAL LOG SHEET

Jan	Feb	Mch	Aprl	May	June	July	Aug	Sept	Oct	Nov	Dec
AN EXAMPLE: Cryostat Temperature Log

The normal range is −20 to −30 degrees centigrade.

(This would be a typical type of daily control chart that you would use for most of the areas of the lab that need daily, 'inspection(s)'). *It is extremely important that these quality control logbooks are maintained and notations made each day that frozen sections are performed. One of the main focuses of an inspection, is proper record keeping.*

SLIDE LABELING

As viewed on an earlier page, I have shown you how all Mohs slides should be labeled. At the top, or 'frosted end,' of the slide you will write patients' *last name first, and first initial. Below that you'll put the Mohs case number, followed by the date. Then below that, the Roman Numeral to denote the 'stage,' of the case. Finally, you will note what piece or part of the section is being cut on the left hand side and the slide number on the right hand side of the slide.*

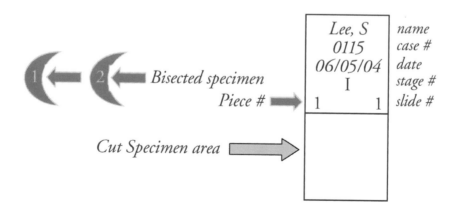

In many offices, the Mohs tech usually knows in advance, the location of the surgical site and the diagnosis. There is a space on your Mohs log-sheet to designate this. Those respective columns would most likely be labeled:

'SITE' – (OR SURGICAL SITE, LOCATION, ETC.)

'DIAGNOSIS' – 99 times out of 100, the diagnosis will either be written out completely or it will be abbreviated. The two most common forms of skin cancer that I've seen excised, using the Mohs method, is *BASAL CELL CARCINOMA, or BCC and SQUAMOUS CELL CARCINOMA, or SCC.*

'STAGE' – Stages are notated in columns provided and noted in Roman Numerals only.

SAMPLE MOHS LOG SHEET

NAME	DATE	CASE#	DIAGNOSIS	SITE	STAGE I	II	III	IV
SMITH J	5\20\04	0165	BCC	TIP OF NOSE	1	1		

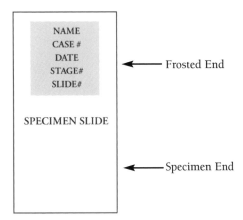

NAME
CASE #
DATE
STAGE#
SLIDE#

SPECIMEN SLIDE

← Frosted End

← Specimen End

Slides are stored in their respective folders for a minimum of one week. This will allow the 'mounting medium,' to harden and dry. Storing the slides prematurely will definitely become one of your worst nightmares when, or if that case requires review, or is requested for review by an inspector. The slides will be stuck together and will have to be soaked for days, before you'll be able to separate them.

When filing the slides, precede each days' work with a paper or precut paper tab, noting the date and the case numbers that are being filed for that day.

Please remember, that when making an entry for each stage that you're cutting, be sure to only note the number of pieces that you have received from the surgeon…not how many pieces you've cut the specimen in to.

Those types of notations only tend to cause confusion and many Inspectors may say that notating what you've done to the specimen is redundant. Don't forget, the surgeon that has excised the tumor has the 'map,' that is drawn, with each succeeding stage.

In closing this chapter, let me emphasize again, the importance of entering all information correctly.

QUESTIONS:

Using the sample Mohs log sheet chart the information given below:

PT. # 1 John Smith—Diagnosis: BCC, 2 stages, Left ear, Case # 0136. When you receive stage I, it is already bisected. when you get stage II, you receive one piece of Tissue.

PT. #2 Susan Jones—Diagnosis: SCC, 3 stages, Tip of nose, Case# 0324. In this case, when you receive stage 1, the doctor has given you one specimen and says to you, 'Bisect it please.' When he hands you stage II, it is also one piece, but he says embed it as it is. When you get stage III, it need no dissecting, so it's embedded as is.

PT. #3 Juan Diaz—Diagnosis: BCC, 4 stages. in this case, when you received your first stage, the surgeon had already dissected the specimen into 4 pieces. when you received stage II, he handed you 2 pieces and in stages III and IV, he gave you one piece each.

MAPPING AND INKING

These next steps are also <u>absolutely critical</u>. So much so, that an error on your part, will lead the Mohs surgeon to believe (assuming the specimen contains tumor) that an area that could have possibly been *free* of tumor, now shows involvement. This of course would require the surgeon to *re-excise* that area of *suspected* involvement, causing the patients' defect to become larger than necessary because the area of the specimen that the doctor had *assumed* contained tumor, is now actually in a different position, than where he thought it was supposed to be. So there is the possibility that a patient that is assumed to be tumor free, isn't.

So… correct orientation is the first step that requires your undivided attention.

In all my years of working with Mohs Surgeons, the specimen is usually handed to you in a variety of different ways: on a piece of gauze, that may have a line drawn directly on it, showing you where '12:00,' is, or the specimen is placed in a petri dish with a gauze pad inside of it, marked with a line, or, you may even receive a,'scaled down,' drawing of the patients' surgical site, with a line drawn, showing you where, '12:00,' is. Look at the specimen as you would imagine the hours on a clock.

Many Mohs surgeons put a, 'knick, or hash mark,' directly on the specimen, so that *there is never a doubt where the 12:00 point of the tissue is.* The shape of the specimen doesn't matter. The surgeon will *always show you his/her orientation point, with a line or arrow.*

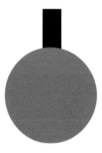

In many cases, you will find that the specimens' shape will vary: the doctor may give you

a round shaped piece

an, oval or ellipitically shaped piece

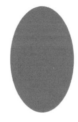

a square or rectangular piece, or a even triangular piece of tissue.

There are always exceptions, but by and large, these are the most common shapes that you'll encounter. The next situation that tends to arise is the, 'thickness of the specimen'.

What many of these types of specimens have in them is a fat layer. Fat is more difficult to cut because it doesn't, 'freeze,' as well and because fat cells retain more water. If there is <u>tumor</u> in the fat layer, it usually <u>will</u> cut and that part of the specimen will be evident in the section. This will be covered in the, 'cryotomy,' section of this manual.

MOST COMMON INK COLORS

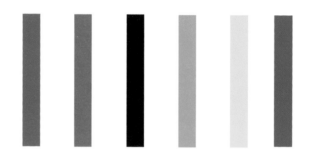

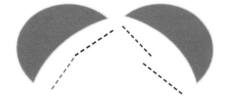

Inked Specimen

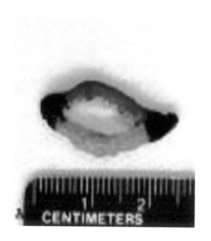

Here's a real one..;)

A Map

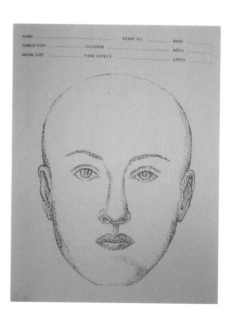

QUESTIONS:

1. Your doctor has given you the first case of the day. This lesion is on the patient's forehead and measures 3.0 cm in length by 1.5 cm in width. He has told you to ink the margins using four colors

Red for 9:00-12:00, Blue for the 12:00-3:00 margin, Yellow for the 3:00-6:00 margin and Black for 6:00-9:00.

2. Today is not your day at work and you drop the patient's' specimen, losing it's orientation. Describe how you would determine the correct orientation of the specimen.

3. As you can see from the colors used for inking specimens, it is very important to remember that when some colors blend together they make another color. Which two colors blended would make the color green?

DISSECTING AND PREPARING THE SPECIMEN FOR EMBEDDING

The problem you must overcome when embedding a specimen, is to try and embed the tissue in such a way, as to insure that the 'skin edge, and the 'deep margin,'are cut by the knife at the same time. 'Splaying,' the specimen (placing thin cuts on various parts of the specimen, to 'relax, the skin edge), or dissecting the specimen are the techniques used, to achieve the desired effect.

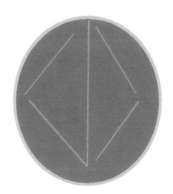

Splaying the Specimen

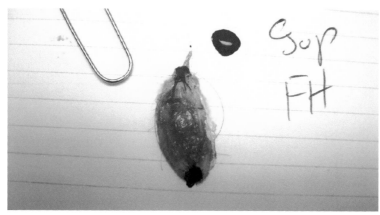

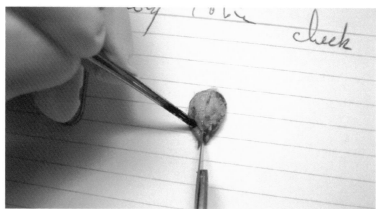

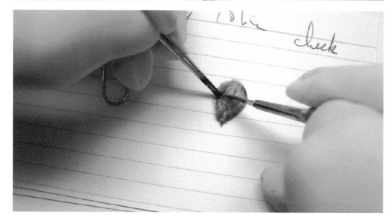

INTRODUCTION TO MOHS CRYOTOMY

You will find many surgeons that will give you the specimen already bisected into two (2) or more pieces. How the 'margins,' are colored is determined by the physician. So, once he has shown you how he likes his 'margins,' inked, it will rarely, if ever, change.

In <u>dissecting</u> (cutting into multiple parts,) or <u>bisecting</u> a specimen, (cutting the tissue in half) maintaining tissue orientation is always focused on before an incision through the specimen is made.

You may find that the specimen given to you by the surgeon you work for, prefers the specimen to be divided/dissected into four (4) quadrants. To do this, you would make a cut with your scalpel, from the 12:00 to the 6:00 axis and another cut with your scalpel, from the 9:00 margin to your 3:00 margin.

Most Mohs surgeons use anywhere from two (2) colors to as many five(5) different ink colors to designate the various margins of the tissue. Many times, if you apply too much ink, it will over power the specimen and hide the most pertinent areas of the tissue that the surgeon needs to see, when viewing the specimen under the microscope. So <u>use the ink sparingly</u>. A little goes a long way. Dab the tissue with a piece of gauze, to wipe off any excess.

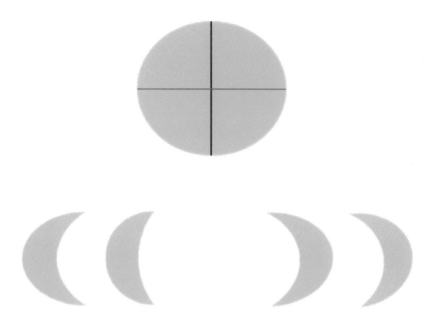

As you can see on the previous page, each piece is inked with two colors. The photo on page 20 is inked with four colors. This of course, aids in pinpointing the location of any area of the specimen that may still contain tumor. A 'positive,' area of the specimen will be re-excised and the same process will begin again. Another point to make here is this: all Mohs surgeons ink their specimens differently, so I can't tell you that there are any hard fast rules in this area. It will take you no time at all, to adapt to another surgeons' style, once you've done a few cases with him. If you're 'lucky,' enough to get some <u>huge</u> tumor to deal with,) the surgeon will give you a description or map of how he wants the specimen inked and dissected. Again, this all stresses the need for you pay close attention and focus when working in a Mohs surgery environment.

QUESTIONS:

This specimen was just handed to you by your surgeon. It is rather large and he tells you to handle it in whatever way is easiest for you. Remember that your chuck may only be about the size of a 25 cent piece. The measurements of this specimen are: 4.0cm x 2.7cm.

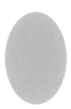

1. First, draw and describe how you're going to splay and then disect the specimen. What entry will you put in your MOHS log for that stage.

TRUE OR FALSE

2. Dividing a specimen in half is the same as saying your're *dissecting* the specimen._____

3. Gently cutting *into* but not *through* a specimen is known as splaying._____

4. The deep margin of the specimen is the least important area of the specimen._____

5. Splaying is one technique used to help relax the skin edge, before embedding._____

EMBEDDING THE PATIENT SPECIMEN

Here comes that word **critical** again. *How* the patients' specimen is embedded, is a concept that many have found difficult to understand.

Let's imagine an orange. Of course, before you eat the orange, you must peel it first. Don't worry, the Mohssurgeon is not peeling the patients' skin off,...;)... But, getting back to that orange. If you were to buy one that had a bruise on it, when you cut through it, you could see how deep or extensive that bruise was. <u>In Mohs surgery, we are not interested as much in how extensive the tumor appears to us on the *surface of the skin, but how extensive the tumor reaches below or underneath the skins' surface.*</u> When thatpatients' specimen is embedded, it is embedded **upside down**. Put another way, the skin surface is embedded face-down, <u>so that the deepest part of the specimen is cut *first*</u>.

In the event you do, by some remote chance forget or remember what you've done until the surgeon reads the slide(s), don't be afraid to tell them. Trust me, if they find out then, if there are consequences, it will only be because of the mistake you made and it will be relatively a minor incident. The important thing is, they know in advance and can either ask you to try and re-embed the specimen correctly, or possibly have you 'cut through it' to find their clear margins that way. Not telling them, means that patient gets excised again, when there is a great chance that the surgeon, 'cleared,' that patient. So, if there's a bone in your body, that is dishonest, or if you don't care about 'accurate documentation,' this job is not for you.

What it WILL do for you, is let your boss know that you're a person of Honor, that takes their job and responsibilities very seriously. Trust between the two of you is vital to your success. Your continued striving to get better, as the time goes by, will also weigh quite posi tively in your Employers' eyes.

Most embedding molds today are made of steel. Steel seems to getcolder faster and also tends to maintain that coldness for a longer period of time.

Here are some of the common embedding molds in use today. Other common types have the same 'post,'that you see, but the embedding surface may be round, instead.See those deep grooves that I was talking about earlier? Those **must be filled with the liquid embedding medium.**

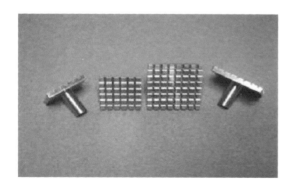

Some Embedding Molds

INTRODUCTION TO **MOHS** CRYOTOMY

The, 'embedding molds,' that are used, vary with the different cryostats that are in use today. Many have a round surface with a thick, 'post,' in the center. Another manufacturers' embedding molds are square, still another manufacturer has square molds too, but their molds come in different sizes.

If you are working in a Mohs surgeons' office and he is contemplating the purchase of a cryostat, we would be more than happy to explain what we feel are the inherent benefits as well as the shortcomings that we've faced, with the different types of cryostats available today.

For some reason, I have found many techs, both experienced as well as inexperienced, making the mistake of placing the embedding molds inside the cryostat, so that they can get, 'cold.' This is a major **NO, NO**. When you examine the various mold configurations that are available today, they all have one thing in common. All have, 'grooves, or indentations,' placed there, so that when the embedding medium is placed on the molds (and when they're at *room temperature*), it has a chance to fill all those spaces. Then, when the medium begins to freeze, it fills all of those spaces *first*. That gives the embedding medium a way for it to, 'anchor,' itself to the mold as it freezes. If you follow this method, you will rarely, if ever, 'pop,' a specimen from it's mold or, 'chuck.'

So don't forget…embedding molds should be at room temperature, before adding embedding medium.

QUESTIONS:

1. When preparing your blocks in advance, it is necessary that they be at room temperature, so that the embedding medium seeps through all of the crevices, during the freezing process. Why is this so?

2. MOHS Embedding is unique because we are cutting the deepest areas of the specimen first. Explain the purpose and reason for this method.

EMBEDDING TECHNIQUE

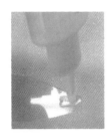

Take a glass slide and put a little mounting medium on the unfrosted end.

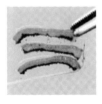

Laying the tissue right side up, we then take the slide and rest it on the cooling bar, inside of the cryostat, gently pressing against the specimen with your Forceps. In moments, it will freeze to the glass slide.

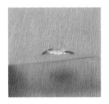

We will then take a chuck that already has embedding medium frozen on it and place one or two drops of liquefied medium on it. Remove the specimen that you have freezing in the cryostat, and _turning the slide upside down_, _gently press the specimen against the chuck, using your index finger. The heat from your finger will enable the specimen to 'slide off,' of the slide, directly on to the chuck._ Take your forceps or scalpel blade to gently tease the skin edge up.

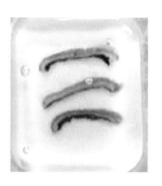

Here is the frozen specimen, embedded on a chuck..

Then, merely return the chuck to the cryostat, cover the specimen with the liquefied mounting medium and gently place your heatextractor over the specimen. Not only will the extractor cool thespecimen faster, it will give you a level 'cutting plane.'

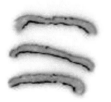

Here is a picture of a _trimmed_ block

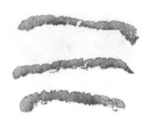

Close up picture of cut and stained slide.

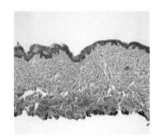

Photomicrograph magnification at 50x

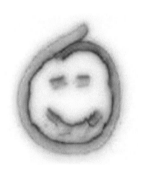

Skin smile, embedded on edge. The skin margin(s) are stained red, the deep margin(s) black.

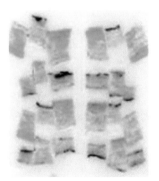

Skin inked and horizontally embedded on edge.

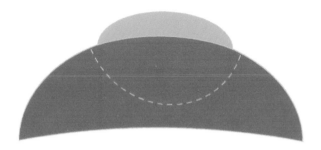

Assume that this diagram is a, 'side view,' of a skin lesion. The blue area lying on the top of the, 'specimen,' is the lesion itself. Looking at the specimen does not tell us whether or not, the tumor goes deep beneath the epidermis (top layer of skin). After we have inked the specimen and are sure of its orientation and have bi or dissected it, we will now **embed the specimen by first turning it upside down**. The diagram below, should help to clarify this for you.

Deep Margin ⟶
Skin Edge ⟶
Lesion ⟶
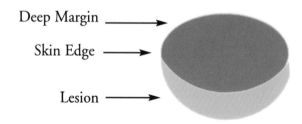

Specimen sitting upside down so that the,'deepest,' layer is facing up.

Now it is time to embed the specimen on the chuck (specimen holder), which already has embedding media frozen on it. Adding a few drops of this room temperature embedding medium to the surface of the chuck, will allow us to place the specimen in such a way, so that we may, 'tease,' the margin(s) up, so that the skin edge and deep margins are cut by the cryostat knife, first. **These very first sections** tell the Mohs surgeon whether or not he has succeeded in removing the entire tumor, when he views your sections under the microscope. Cutting too deeply into the tissue could cause the surgeon to assume that the margins are still involved, causing him to re-excise the area of suspicion.

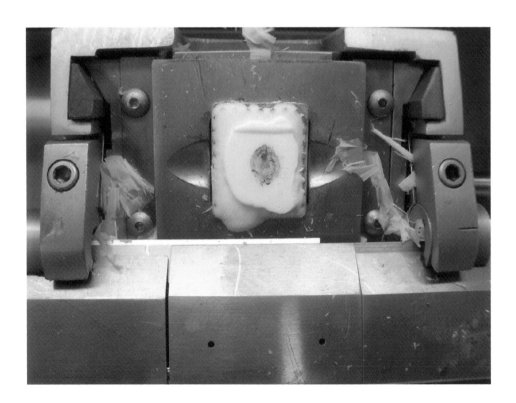

VERTICAL OR HORIZONTAL EMBEDDING

One of the primary reasons that Mohs surgery has such a high cure rate, is due largely in part, to the positioning of the specimen prior to it being cut in the cryostat. In Mohs, all specimens are embedded horizontally. When embedding horizontally, the surgeon gets to see both the deep margin and skin edge, simultaneously. In a verti-cally embedded specimen, the surgeon only gets to see the uppermost layers of the specimen, greatly increasing the chance of missing tumor that could be found deep in the tissue. Below is an attempt at rendering a description of vertical embedding.

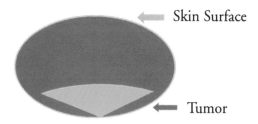

Skin Surface

Tumor

As you can see, when cutting vertically, the tumor could be missed entirely.

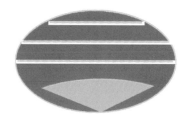

One golden rule I've always followed. Be conservative when you cut these specimens. Once you've cut through it, it's gone forever. If you haven't gone deep enough, the surgeon will tell you and you'll have more than enough specimen left, to give the surgeon more of what he needs to see. If you cut too deeply into the specimen, it could lead to a re-excision of the patient, costing not only the patient, but the surgeon's time, repairing the defect. One more thing: If the surgeon tells you he is not seeing the skin edge, you will need to melt the specimen and reembed, or re-orient your block, then, cut and stain the tissue again.

In closing, embedding Mohs specimens can be done in a variety of ways. There are individuals that have designed, patented and currently sell their embedding systems. All are quite effective in ensuring that he entire specimen is embedded perfectly. You will, with time, select the way(s) that is most effective for you. Until then, keep it simple. Be sure you've splayed the specimen we enough, so that all margins are able to be embedded flat.

QUESTIONS:

1. I have described two basic methods of embedding tissue when doing a Mohs procedure. One of course, is embedding directly onto the frozen embedding mold or chuck. The other technique requires the use of a slide. Explain how you will embed your specimen using the glass slide technique. Also be sure to mention tissue orientation in your explanation.

TRUE OR FALSE

2. When preparing your molds (chucks), they should always be kept inside the cryostat, before you cover them with embedding compound._____

3. The outer skin surface is the most critical part of the specimen that the Mohs surgeon needs to see when viewing your slide.._____

4. Vertical embedding is the method of choice when embedding MOHS skin specimens.._____

5. Place the specimen upside down when embedding from a glass slide._____

6. Vertical embedding enables the surgeon to see both the skin edge and deep marginds of the entire specimen, simultaneously._____

7. When embedding using the glass slide method, the tissue is always placed onto the glass with the deepest margins facing you._____

CRYOTOMY

This phase of the Mohs procedure will take a lot of practice, before you become truly proficient in this area.

There are a number of cryostats on the market today, with many Mohs surgeons using machines that have been out of manufacture for a number of years. You will be trained on the instrument that your surgeon owns. Why the instrument is called a cryostat is simply because the 'microtome,' which actually sections or cuts the tissue, sits inside of a refrigerated cabinet. Let me warn you now, **it gets very, very cold in there**. Remember the film where the young boy sticks his tongue onto a metal pole and gets it stuck there because the pole is so ice cold? The same applies to cryotomy. I don't expect that you will be sticking your tongue in to the interior of the cryostat, but if you'll remember that movie, you'll get the general idea. Cryostat interior temperature(s) range from an average minus 18 to minus 30 degrees Centigrade. Trust me, that is very, very cold!!! So, NO WET HANDS IN THE CRYOSTAT.

Once you've embedded the specimen on the 'chuck,' you will replace it back into the machine, so that the tissue freezes fully.

Any Mohs tech I've ever known, always places their disposable knife and brushes (used for 'teasing,' the specimen) in the cryostat long before the surgical day begins. Try to remember to never leave the entire package of blades in the Cryostat. Upon defrosting, moisture will develop in the dispenser and the blades will begin to rust.

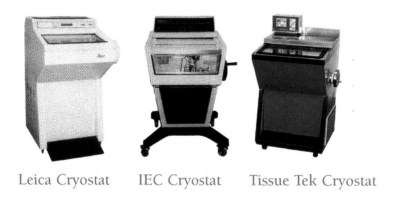

Leica Cryostat   IEC Cryostat   Tissue Tek Cryostat

WORKING WITH BRUSHES

Learning to work with brushes, when performing frozen sections will make your life so much easier. The purpose of the brush is to grab and maneuver the section across the stage. The section is by nature, trying to curl up and pull away from the brush. For this reason I use a brush with stiff bristles and a fairly wide gripping surface. As you can see from this photo, the brush is held like a pen. In this second picture (on the right) you can see the brush, 'teasing or guiding,' the specimen away from the knife. I assume you know what the right-hand most picture is…;)

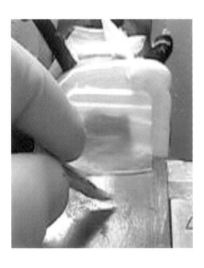

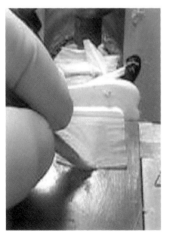

Notice that brush merely guides the tissue away from the knife.Pulling the specimen will cause it to tear

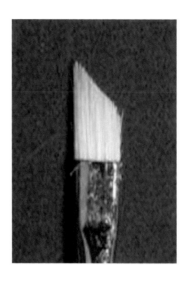

Brush edge trimmed at an angle.

Condensation will cause the blades to rust. Also, when turning off the cryostat for a few days, be sure that it is kept scrupulously clean after each use. It is also a MUST, that you leave the cryostat drawer opened, so that any moisture can evaporate. Built up moisture will turn to ice, making it difficult, if not impossible to cut a section. **Never force** the wheel to turn. Doing so could break the 'teeth,' on the gears of the microtome, making it impossible to cut a section. The cost of repairing something like that could be quite substantial.

I believe that cleaning with alcohol would be your best bet. Be sure it isn't a 'dilute,' alcohol, such as 70%, 80%, etc. <u>100% alcohol</u>, being water free, would be wisest, unless you're turning the cryostat off.. Chemicals like bleach, will eat away at the stainless steel interior.

In getting back to the knives used in a cryostat, there are basically two different types: *disposable blades* and what I'd call '*fixed*,' blades. The great advantage to the disposable blade is simple...when they get dull or have been nicked, they can merely be replaced. Fixed blades are much longer in length, creating a huge risk factor of cutting yourself. These types of blades extend out beyond the holder they're placed in and I know from personal experience, you can really cut yourself, causing quite a bit of damage. The other big drawback to fixed blades is that they require sharpening. Your choices of sharpening leaves you with only two options. Sending them out to a commercial blade manufacturer for 'reconditioning,' or purchasing an automated sharpener. Granted, they work beautifully, but they are expensive and require that you purchase sharpening compounds of varying coarseness. If you've 'nicked,' the blade rather deeply, you'll be forced to send the blade out...meaning more dollars spent, purchasing a sharpener and the need to own a few of these fixed blades. Disposable blades cost an average of $1.00 a piece, come in packs of approximately 50 blades and will last you months and as I said before, when they get dull or nicked, merely throw them away and minutes later, you're ready to cut again. When inserting any type of microtome blade into your cryostat, be *careful*. These blades are <u>amazingly</u> sharp!

KNIFE ANGLE is of utmost importance in determining how your tissue 'cuts.' If the angle is not precise, tissue may 'compress,' or 'bunch up,' on the knife edge, or worse still, you may have difficulty getting a section at all!! No matter what type of blades you use, the manufacturer or seller of the cryostat should be able to tell you what angle to set your knife angle at. Once it's set and you're getting good sections, <u>leave it alone</u>. There could be other reasons why you may be having difficulties getting a good frozen section. Here are some other possibilities: cryostat isn't cold enough-plan on four (4) hours (if you forgot to turn the machine on the night before.) Most machines don't take quite that long, to get to operating temperature, but better 'safe than sorry.' Cutting for a Mohs surgeon can be stressful enough.

Remember this: HEAT CAN BE YOUR WORST ENEMY!!

Also, the rooms' temperature will make a big difference in your ability to get a good section. You're trying to cut tissue at **−24 degrees** centigrade!!!

KNIFE CHATTER: this can be caused by a number of things: your specimen hasn't been tightened in it's holder tightly enough, you've sprayed the specimen so much with your can of 'freeze spray,' that you yourself, could create another ice age...;)making the specimen too cold, you forgot to tighten the knife or it's holder, or you're turning the cryostat wheel so fast, you've created your own tornado! When you receive your 'hands on training,' the possible problems that could arise, will be addressed in detail.

It is most important that the specimen holder, knife holder and the knife itself, be tightened. loose parts will cause chatter,or worse, cause you to chop through the block/specimen.

EXAMPLES OF KNIFE 'CHATTER'

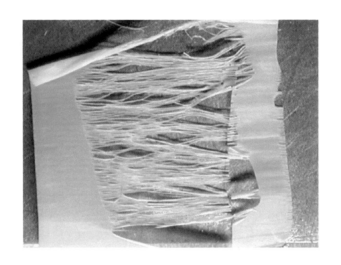

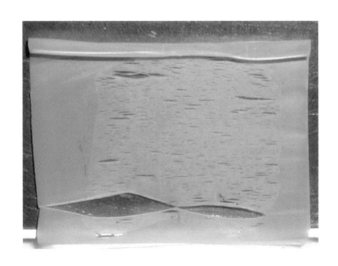

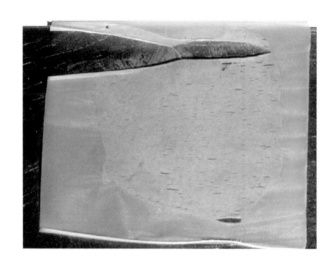

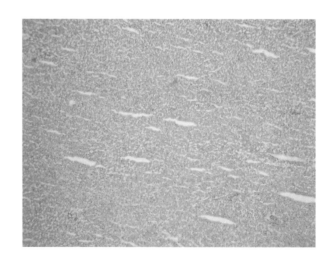

H & E stain of previous photograph.

INTRODUCTION TO **MOHS** CRYOTOMY

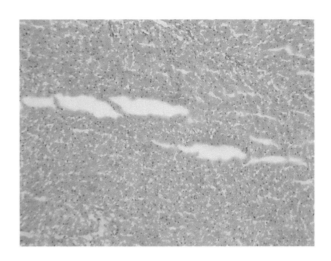

Photomicrographs of knife chatter

QUESTIONS:

1. Give three reasons for knife chatter.

2. Blowing into your cryostat to remove waste sections will cause your sections to curl. Why?

3. Explain what instances may cause tissue compression when cutting your patient's specimen.

4. Leaving your box of cryostat blades inside the instrument will ruin your

blades after time. Why?

5. What would you consider to be a good cryostat operating temperature, when cutting skin specimens?

6. Using large amounts of freeze spray on a specimen just prior to cutting it could cause what kind of an effect?

7. In the event that someone neglected to turn the cryostat on the night before surgeries, you can assume that the average amount of time the instrument will need to reach operating temperature is approximately_____ hours.

CUTTING TECHNIQUE

The greatest histotech in the world, would be unable to describe in words, the techniques for getting a good result from the specimen you're trying to cut. Remember ano-ther thing…you just so happen to be trying to take a slice of that specimen so thin, it's thinner than a sheet of paper!! To be more precise, when that tissue 'comes off,' of the knife edge, that section is approximately five (5) twenty five thousandths (25,000th) of an inch thick!!! The one on one training you'll get, will help you understand more. I mentioned '*brushes*,' earlier. Some techs prefer camel hair brushes (that you'd buy at any crafts store), others like synthetic ones and some even use wooden applicator sticks. The preference is totally up to you. As I said before, practice, is what will make you good at cutting frozen sections. The reason for these brushes is this: it helps you 'guide,' or 'tease,' the section as it comes off of the knife edge. By *very gently* guiding the section from the knife you will be able to guide (hopefully), without tearing, the specimen. With practice, you'll be even able to tease out wrinkles and flatten skin edges, if necessary.

TYPES AND CUTTING CHARACTERISTICS OF VARIOUS TYPES OF TISSUE

How fortunate for you, that you've decided to make the cutting of 'skin,' a priority. Skin itself is relatively easy to cut by frozen section. As mentioned before, *horizontal embedding*, is what makes this technique unique because it gives the surgeon the 'whole picture,' when the specimen is embedded FLAT.

Tissue orientation, when you're ready to cut, is also of prime importance. Having the skin edge angled at approximately a 70 degree angle, or perpendicular to the knife edge is critical. You may experience 'curling,' of the skin edge that touches the knife edge first, but working on your 'brush,' technique, will help you greatly. Having the tissue parallel to the knife will only cause you tremendous aggravation!!

Your next biggest problem is dealing with 'fatty,' specimens. As mentioned earlier, fat is very difficult to cut. Some suggestions on how to deal with specimens like that, is a challenge at best. Here are a few that might make cutting the fat easier for you.

Fat should be the last thing to hit the blade or should hit the blade by itself when possible. Fat does not get hard enough to cut well at temperatures that are best for cutting most other tissues. When fat hits the blade before the more manageable tissues, it may smear and ruin the rest of the section. I find, that by hitting the knife last or by itself, fat won't interfere with the other tissues as much. If I find myself having difficulty getting a good section because fat appears in the plane, I suggest rotating the chuck to avoid the fat. Another suggestion: keep a *canister of liquid nitrogen* on hand. You think the cryostat gets cold? All Dermatologists' use liquid nitrogen to 'freeze,' certain types of skin conditions on the patients they see. So, spraying a little of the nitrogen *only on the fatty portion* of the specimen will help greatly. Make sure that your blade is either new, or moved to an unused portion, that it is clean and that the stage is wiped clean, as well.

Avoid having the fat hit the blade first if possible. The fat will pull away from the embedding medium and start a hole. If a little non fatty tissue is next to the embedding medium it gives it a little better bind to the medium and a better start to the section.

Here is where the clean swift turn of the wheel without hesitation is most important.

If the tissue is a mixture of fat and connective tissues it will cut better than pure fat. Sometimes, surprisingly well, if you follow all of the techniques I have mentioned. Catch the edge of the tissue in motion and quickly and pull the section across the stage with the brush. Do not press the brush and tissue against the stage. It will stick and you won't be able to cut anything until you clean it. A good sharp blade will help. If you can make this swift cut you will be able to get reasonable sections of some fairly fatty tissues. The fat may appear as large empty spaces but the fibrous strands between them will be cut well.

Always lock the wheel when placing or removing a specimen from the object holder. The blade is only millimeters from your fingers and the last thing you

want, is to cut yourself with a blade you've been using on a patient.

You may find that a specimen is too cold, or for the reasons mentioned earlier, you may experience 'knife chatter.' Placing your thumb on the specimen for a moment should help in resolving that problem. Taking thicker sections can be a good adjunct to reading your best attempt at a thin section. Thicker sections can be made in a variety of ways. On my automated cryostat I first try with a single press of the fine advance button. If conservation of tissue is not an issue I may try a very quick press of the course advance. This will produce a very thick section. You can also adjust the section thickness dial or take a double click of the wheel by cranking forward a quarter turn, then backward , and again forward. This variety of maneuvers will produce a range of section thickness. If you then turn the wheel in a continuous very deliberate fashion while using your best brush technique, you can end up with a slice of butter to pick up on the slide. Be very gentle with the tissue in the solutions. No vigorous movements. You certainly don't want your best efforts washing off of the slide. 'Treated,' slides, fixation and even gentle heat, will help insure that your sections remain on the slide..

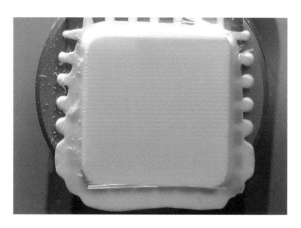

Wavy lines "Chatter"

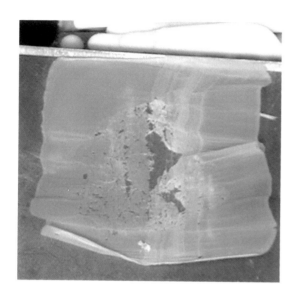

Tissue adhering to the underside of the blade.

QUESTIONS:

1. Orientation of the specimen is most important when cutting frozen sections. The skin edge should always be _____to the knife edge.

2. Describe the reasoning behind embedding MOHS skin sections horizontally.

3. On the previous page you see a section that demonstrates 'Knife Chatter.' Give three reasons why that happened.

4 You've received a very faty specimen and the surgeon tells you how important it is that he see the entire section. What steps can you take to ensure that he sees the fatty area of the specimen?

5. Explain the main reason that vertical embedding should never be used when cutting a MOHS frozen section.

6. You're preparing to cut this specimen. What problems (if any) will you have obtaining a good section of this specimen? (Hint: This question is asking about tissue orientation.)

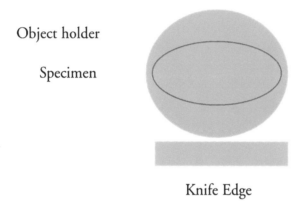

Object holder

Specimen

Knife Edge

7. When you are using your brushes, you notice that the specimen is tearing as you guide it away from the knife. What could cause that?

8. Describe a method for cutting fatty specimens.

THE 'X/Y' AXIS

If you refer back a few pages to the picture of some of the various models of cryostats being used today, the instrument on the extreme right, does not have this feature. The X/Y axis, simply put, enables you to re-orient your embedded block, in the event that one part of the tissue is being cut more deeply or unevenly than another. The advantage, of course, is that you can re-orient your embedded block, so that the features in the specimen that the knife is 'missing,' you'll be able to cut. If you're working with a machine like the one on the right, proper embedding is essential.

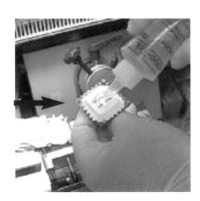

Just behind that bottle of embedding medium is the handle and knob that you use to adjust the chuck angle.

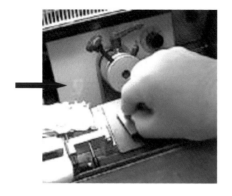 Here is a slightly better picture of the chuck, its handle and knob.

MICROSCOPE SLIDES

There are countless brands and varieties of slides available today. The most important point is that they be 'frosted,' so that you can write the pertinent information on them with an **indelible pen**. When I refer to 'frosted,' the slide has one area that takes up about one quarter of the total length of the slide, which is coarser and/or colored, so that you can write on them.

Some slides are 'pre-coated,' with a substance that will help adhere the section to the slide. I've used both the 'coated,' as well as uncoated slides. The difference in cost is unbelievable. Coated slides are extremely expensive. If you will look at the sections on the following page, you may be able to note the difference in clarity and 'crispness,' of the cells on the sections that were fixed, prior to being stained.

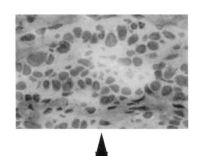

Specimen after 15 Min. drying time

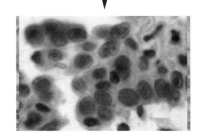

Same tissue immediately fixed in 95% Alcohol

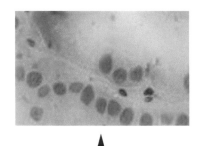

Another specimen after 15 min. drying Time.

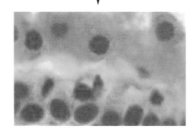

Same specimen imme-diately fixed in 95% Alcohol

If you 'fix,'the specimen, that should help considerably and save the expense of 'coated,' slides.

FIXING THE SPECIMEN TO THE SLIDE

I personally prefer the type(s) of fixatives that can legally be disposed of, down the sink. The other main purpose of a fixative, is to prevent 'autolysis' or cell death. The surgeon will get much better 'morphological,' detail, if the slides are fixed, before they are stained. The quicker you can get nice sections on a slide and get the slide fixed, the better.

Fixatives like formalin, which is made from Formaldehyde, have a number of issues: it's a suspected carcinogen and the fumes are toxic. In most states that lie on bodies of water, it's illegal to pour it down the sink and your surgeons' laboratory is responsible for it from day of receipt until day of disposal. Finding honest, reliable waste disposal companies can be a challenge. The actual term is this:

QUESTIONS:

1. Using the Photomicrographs above, describe the benefits of slide fixation.

2. The X/Y axis offers one great improvement in cryotomy. Explain its features and benefits.

3. Describe the main purposes of fixation.

4. Slide fixation prevents_____.

CRADLE TO GRAVE LIABILITY
AND THE H & E STAIN

It's your responsibility, from the moment you receive these chemicals until it has been disposed of, properly. If that hauler you've hired is caught dumping your waste in an unapproved area…the government goes after your boss and he pays. Needless to say, toxic chemicals have no place in a private laboratory. The other alternatives, besides Alcohol as a fixative, are the fixatives made by various lab suppliers. These are marketed specifically to fit the need of making readily disposable, non-toxic chemicals for use in laboratories.

STAINING The reason that we 'stain,' the tissue is because microscopically, tissue is basically colorless. It is part of our job as Mohs techs, to give the tissue color, so that the surgeon can make his diagnosis. The most common stain used today is called the 'H & E,' stain. The H, standing for Hematoxylin, a stain that used to be made from tree bark and the E, standing for 'Eosin,' a synthetic stain that dyes everything. We use these stains and a series of other reagents to produce stained sections the surgeon can 'read.'

FIX the slide (previously discussed) for a few moments in 95% alcohol.

RINSE fixative off of slide(s) with gently running water.

HEMATOXYLIN When placing slides in stain (1'30" is good) agitate the slide(s) gently when you place them in the stain. This will help insure even staining. Hematoxylin is a wonderful 'nuclear stain'.

Rinse until water runs clear.

BLUE This water based substance helps to enhance the staining characteristics of Hematoxylin and you will actually see the tissue turn bluer..

Rinse Be sure to rinse the slides well. Some bluing reagents will fade the stain(s) in time.

95% REAGENT ALCOHOL This 'sets,' up the tissue for the next step, Eosin. There are different schools of thought whether one should go directly from water into Eosin, or my way of staining, which would include this step first.

EOSIN This is a reddish colored, synthetic stain that stains all parts of the tissue. Diluted reagent alcohol will remove the excess stain from the parts of the tissue that we don't need stained with Eosin. This is a wonderful stain for 'cytoplasm'.

95% REAGENT ALCOHOL; The purpose of a 'diluted,' alcohol *immediately following* the Eosin, is for removing some of the excess stain. If you'll note earlier, I mentioned that Eosin is a 'cytoplasmic stain, but.... it stains every part of the tissue. So, by adding water to the alcohol, we are making a 'dilution,' of the reagent. Dilutions are made quite simply, by multiplying the percent solution you want, (in this case, 95% alcohol) by 100. Since we're dealing with percentages, multiply the 100 X .95. You should come up with 95, leaving you with 5, left over, to make the 95% . That '5' would represent cc's or ml's. In this case, we're diluting with water, so 5 cc's of water would be added to the 95 cc's of alcohol, giving you 100cc of a 95% solution of alcohol.. In the medical field, most measurements are done using the'metric system.' Liquids, metrically speaking, are described either in'cc's,' or in '**ml's**. CC stands for cubic centimeters and ML stands for milliliters.

100% REAGENT ALCOHOL This helps to remove any more excess Eosin and water that may still be on the specimen slide(s). I would recommend three (3) changes of 100% alcohol, before going into any type of 'clearing,' solution.

CLEARING SOLUTION In many larger laboratories a petroleum based chemical known as xylene is still used. It probably is, one of the finest 'clearing,' reagents there is, but it too, is toxic, wreaks havoc on your skin, the fumes are very intense and it is also highly flammable. This chemical, like Formalin, must be disposed of legally, by hiring a licensed waste hauler. There are some more than adequate clearing solutions available today, that are not toxic, practically odorless, easy on the skin and best of all, can be poured down the sink.

Many techs will have a separate container with clean clearing solution in it, before they will coverslip.

By the time you've come to this step, the slides should be totally dehydrated (all water removed.) The clearing agent is miscible,' (able to mix with) with alcohol and if by chance, you should see globules of water when you're rinsing in clearant, (just like you'd see at home, if you added water to cooking oil) then you probably have contamination in your last 100% alcohol. When first dipping into the first clearant , you'll see a 'syrupy,' appearance on the slides. As you continue to dip them, that should start to disappear, certainly by the second change of clearant and by the third change, you should see nothing, but your *beautiful* sections, that you'll now:

MOUNT AND COVERSLIP- Mounting medium is merely a clear liquid, hard drying adhesive, that helps to adhere the coverslip to the slide. When done properly, there are no 'air bubbles,' trapped beneath the coverglass and that will guarantee you that your slides will remain perfectly preserved for years to come.

It seems like we all have our own 'tricks,' for coverslipping our slides. Some lay the slides down, putting the liquified mounting medium on the lower part of the slide, then butting the coverslip to the slides' edge, gently lowering it onto the specimen slide. Others hold the slide, adding a few drops of mounting media at the bottom of the slide and let 'capillary action,' take the medium from one end of the slide to the other before allowing the coverslip to cover the entire speci-men.

As I mentioned earlier, it is essential that the slides be given time to dry. Wiping off any excess when you're initially coverslipping will help too. There's nothing more aggravating to the surgeon than to have to continually wipe his microscope stage, because excess mounting media and clearant are smearing all over the place.

In time, as the mounting medium bottle is opened, the medium tends to get very 'viscous.' Simply put, viscosity describes how 'thick, or syrupy, the mounting media is getting. As the weeks go by, it will get more and more syrupy, making mounting of your coverslip more difficult. Try and keep the bottle loosely closed, in between uses. Many times, if you'll just add an extra drop of clean clearing agent to the slide, that will thin the mounting media just enough, so that you're able to coverslip your slide with the minimum amount of difficulty.

Another *very important point*: all mounting mediums are not the same and you must be sure that it is compatible with the Clearing agent you are using. If not, your slides will fade with time and the longer that slide has had time to dry, the harder and longer it will take you to remove that coverslip, praying at all times, that when you do get the coverslip off, that it doesn't take any of the sections off with it.

QUESTIONS:

1. Since Hematoxylin is a water based stain,the step that always *precedes* immersion in Hematoxylin is _____

2. When liquids are able to be absorbed by one another, you could also say that they are_____.

3. If you find 'Globules,' in your clearing agent,what is the most likely containment?_____.

4. What step is necessary in order to 'Blue,' the tissue when stsaining?

5. What chemical helps to reduce the intensity of Eosin?

6. If you and your boss elect touse Formalin and/or Xylene, these chemicals must be disposed off properly. In many states your responsibility for these chemicals begins, when you take possession of them. The term used for this is known as_____.

MICROSCOPE

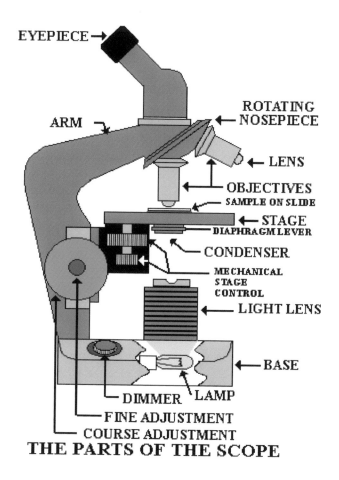

EYEPIECE →

ARM

ROTATING NOSEPIECE ←

← LENS

OBJECTIVES

SAMPLE ON SLIDE

← STAGE

DIAPHRAGM LEVER

CONDENSER

MECHANICAL STAGE CONTROL

LIGHT LENS ←

← BASE

DIMMER ─ LAMP

FINE ADJUSTMENT

COURSE ADJUSTMENT

THE PARTS OF THE SCOPE

As you will learn, if you're not already aware, the microscope is key in the surgeons' ability to make his diagnosis.

Treat this instrument with the utmost respect. Never clean any of the lenses with anything other than 'lens paper.' Be sure to keep the microscope covered when not in use. Dust particles or worse, scratches, look HUGE when magnified 5, 10, 40 or even 100 times. I will not go into the various parts and their functions here. Your need for the microscope is simple: you merely want to be sure that the sections that you've cut and stained, show all of the necessary parts of the specimen that you've received. Is the skin edge present, in toto? Are you able to see your 'inked,' margins? Have you cut into the section deeply enough (careful, not too deep), so that everything the surgeon needs to see, is present? If not and you're quick enough, you may be able to cut him another few sections, get it stained and coverslipped, so that when the doctor sees the slides, you've saved yourself, the patient and the surgeon, the time of having to wait for you to cut and process more sections.

RECORD KEEPING

As I said in the very beginning of this manual, record keeping is certainly one of the most important aspects of this kind of work. Compliance with County, State and Federal Regulations are an absolute necessity. The accuracy of your record keeping puts a considerable amount of responsibility on you. As I mentioned earlier, Inspectors want to see that every 'I,' is dotted and every 'T,' is crossed. I can't imagine an inspector from ANY government agency, tolerating slipshod, sloppy, inaccurate, or illegible documentation. Fraudulent records can cost you dearly. It can be very, very intimidating when Agency vehicles and trucks pull up to the office, send all patients home and sequester each employee into a private room and question them until 1am in the morning. When you see men with hand trucks carting off almost all of the doctors' patient files, to be scrutinized by accountants, medicare agents and/or the FBI, I promise you, it's a very serious matter.

So, by keeping everything YOU do, as accurate and perfect as possible, you'll be the one leaving with your head held high, knowing that nothing you did can hurt you or the physician you are working for.

It's also a wonderful feeling when your boss comes to you after an inspection and the laboratory that you're responsible for has no violations or citations. Believe me, Mohs surgery is growing by leaps and bounds every year and word gets out, a tmeetings, symposiums, etc. Let your boss spread the word to his colleagues, describing how lucky he/she is to have a Mohs tech so dedicated to *their* work, as he/she is dedicated to their profession.

Again, make your entries each day that Mohs surgery is performed. If you've had an instrument serviced or repaired…or you've had trouble with a stain and you've changed the staining lineup or protocol, make sure that you've noted it. Save all receipts and documentation from repairmen, installers of equipment, warranty work, etc., and keep it on file in the same books that you keep your 'quality control,' logbooks.

Your accuracy, your abilities at being meticulous in your work and your desire to be great at what you do will take you very far in this field.

I promise you, that the day will come when you will have a great sense of satisfaction every day that you cut frozens, because you'll know that the part you played in clearing the patient was directly related to your skill(s)as a Mohs Histotech.

EQUIPMENT MAINTENANCE

I guess it's needless to say, that maintaining the instruments that you use, will make your life much, much easier. Your cryostat, regardless of what brand or make it is, requires scrupulous cleaning after each use, as well as lubrication. NEVER, I repeat, NEVER, leave a knife blade in the holder of the cryostat. Too many accidents have occurred because of this oversight. As I mentioned earlier, if you're not doing Mohs on a daily basis, turn the machine off and keep the glass door opened!!!

Make sure that you filter your Hematoxylin and Eosin before each day begins. Cells from previous specimens tend to slough off of slides and you wouldn't want your boss telling you that he sees 'cross-contamination,' on your slides, or water globules trapped under the coverslip because you were too lazy to change the reagents that day.

We have already briefly discussed the microscope. As a part of your training, we will go through the steps involved in keeping it in top condition.

All of the instruments that you use in the Mohs lab are quite costly and the way you maintain and care for your doctors' equipment is just another reflection of how you view your job and responsibilities. When you have completed this course of training, you will be fairly proficient in this line of work and will have the confidence of knowing that you received the most intensive course of study available for Mohs Cryotomy.

You have my sincerest wishes for your success in pursuing this most exciting and rewarding career. You all have my address and telephone number. I'll be happy to discuss, help, or troubleshoot any difficulties you may have, along the way.

ACKNOWLEDGEMENT

In closing, I would like to thank Dr. Stephen Peters, M.D. of Pathology Innovations, LLC, Hackensack, New Jersey…for his generosity in allowing me use of some of his material. When I spoke with him over the telephone, I found a true kindred spirit. I too believe that Mohs Cryotomy is a science of course, but it is also what we both consider to be an art form.

ABOUT THE AUTHOR

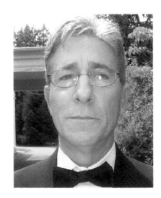 Upon graduating Laboratory Technology training in New York City, Mr. Lee moved to Florida where he began his work in Histology. Mr. Lee worked for one of the first Mohs Surgeons in Palm Beach County in 1982 and has continued working in that specialty for a number of surgeons in the South Florida region. This past year, Mr. Lee created the first employment Staffing Agency that specifically address this most specific area of expertise. www.mohstechstaffing.com is a website designed to place qualified Mohs Techs with Mohs Surgeons. In addition, Mr. Lee also offers individual and group training programs